SURVIVING A BURNOUT

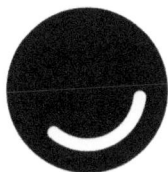

ISBN: 978-978-61039-4-5

Published in Nigeria by WORITAL GLOBAL, 2024
6b Lanre Awolokun Street, Gbagada Phase 2, Lagos, Nigeria.
WORITAL (hello@worital.com)
+2348114027024

Interior Layout, Print and Bound by:
WORITAL (hello@worital.com)

WORITAL
Dream . Work . Achieve

Dedication

This book is a testament to the love, support, and encouragement I received during one of the most challenging phases of my life. Undoubtedly, I would not have been able to reclaim my well-being and get my life back on track without the incredible people who stood by me.

Therefore, to my lovely wife, Ehi, and my son, Weyinmi—your constant love and patience have been one of my greatest wells of strength. Both of you have been my rock, and I am forever grateful for your presence in my life.

My heartfelt gratitude goes to these people: My dear sister, Mrs. Maureen Ebigbeyi, and family, General Ochigbano, and his wife, Mrs. Eunice Ochigbano—your kindness and support have been a reservoir of comfort and strength.

A special thanks to Dr. Edward Oladele, Dr. Eluke Francis, and Dr. Felicia Meriga; your guidance and wisdom have been invaluable, and your support and belief in me during those difficult times have been a beacon of hope.

These individuals also played a significant role in my recovery and I am extending my deepest gratitude to them: Mrs. Christy Laniyan, Dr. Hadiza Khamofu, Mr. Audu Amushe, and the staff of FHI 360. Your encouragement and understanding were a much-needed lifeline during those moments when I thought my life would never be the same.

I wouldn't trade your friendship for anything: Ope Abiodore, Bridget Nwagbara, Ada Umolu-Okeke, Andy Omoluabi, and family—thank you for your constant support and for being there when I needed it most. Your friendship has been a true blessing to me.

I am also deeply grateful to Rev. Fr. Francis Mario, Rev. Fr. Andrew Sule, and Rev. Fr. Joseph Akande; your spiritual guidance and prayers have provided me with resilience and helped me dare greatly to overcome those challenges I faced.

To my elder brother, Emmanuel "Tunde" Etsetowaghan and his family, the entire Odagbali and Etsetowaghan families, and the FGC Warri Class of '93—your unwavering support during my trying phase has been truly priceless, and I'm eternally grateful.

To the people in my Abuja Chaingang Cycling family, you have proved to be a second family. I appreciate your support and kindness through visits and phone calls because they were instrumental to my recovery.

If you were a part of my recovery journey, whether or not you are mentioned here, please know that I am deeply grateful to you for supporting me during that difficult time, and this book reflects the strength that I drew from each of you.

Acknowledgment

Introduction of Contributors to
'Surviving a Burnout'

The creation of *Surviving a Burnout* has been enriched by the profound experiences and insights of three incredible individuals who shared their personal and professional perspectives on overcoming burnout.

Dr. Bridget Nwagbara, a public health expert and burnout survivor, brings a unique perspective based on her own experience with the pressures of healthcare leadership and birth.

Her experience as a healthcare professional and a survivor provides readers with a deeply relatable story of resilience, strength, and indomitable spirit, as well as the strategies she used to reclaim her health.

Dr. Sam Abah, a distinguished psychiatrist, provides expert insight into the psychological dimensions of burnout. His contributions to the book focus on the challenges of managing mental health disorders while navigating the corridors of associated stigma and socio-cultural beliefs.

Finally, we have **Rev. Father Andrew Sule**, a Catholic priest, who adds a spiritual viewpoint to the discussion of burnout. In his reflections on faith, inner peace, and the importance of spiritual well-being, Father Sule provides a holistic approach to recovery, reminding readers of the value of purpose and the strength that comes from within during difficult times.

Together, these contributors give a comprehensive and compassionate guide to navigating burnout, while blending personal stories with a touch of professional expertise in order to help readers not only survive but thrive through life's toughest challenges unscathed.

Contents

Introduction

THE SILENT
STORM OF BURNOUT

In the hushed moments of early dawn, when the world is
still and calm, I often find myself reflecting on the years
I spent navigating the turbulent waters of burnout. It was
like a storm brewing slowly until it became overwhelming and
threatened to take away everything I cared about—my passion,
health, and relationships.

As I write this, I am reminded of the days when I would wake
up feeling like a shadow of my former self, each task ahead
resembling an insurmountable mountain and every interaction
leaving me drained. I used to be a person who believed strongly
in pursuing one's goals and was an unwavering believer in the
power of hard work, but amidst my achievements and successes,
I lost my sense of 'self'.

The tiredness that crept in turned into a loud shout, and the bright colors of my life faded to grey. I had a firsthand experience of the physical and emotional toll of burnout—those nights spent staring at the ceiling, wrestling with anxiety and guilt, and wondering where the spark of joy had gone.

This book is not merely a collection of research and statistics; it is a personal story of my journey through the labyrinth of burnout and the lessons I learned along the way.

I invite you to walk with me as I share the moments that catalyzed my awakening, the strategies I employed to reclaim my life, and the insights gained from countless conversations with others who have faced the same silent adversary. Together, we will explore the complexities of burnout—the societal pressures that fuel it, the stigma surrounding it, and the paths to healing that lie ahead.

It is my hope that through these pages, you will find not only validation for your struggles but also the tools and inspiration to rise from the ashes of burnout. Whether you are currently trapped in its grasp or seeking to prevent its onset, this journey is for you—a testament to resilience, self-discovery, and the profound importance of nurturing our well-being.

As we embark on this exploration, let us remember that while burnout may be a formidable adversary, it is not insurmountable.

Together, we can reclaim our lives, ignite our passions anew, and rediscover the joy that lies within.

Chapter One

THE BEGINNING OF THE END

"Sometimes to live is an act of courage."
- Lucius Annaeus Seneca

Bisoprolol Fumarate is a drug that was first discovered and patented in 1976 and approved for medical use in 1986, the year I was born. It is used for cardiovascular diseases, including high blood pressure (hypertension), angina, and heart failure.

If you have high blood pressure, taking Bisoprolol helps prevent future heart disease, heart attacks, and strokes. It works by slowing down your heart rate and making it easier for your heart to pump blood around your body. Basically, the drug attempts to stop the heart from committing suicide. The cardiologist said, "If you don't slow down, your heart might not stand the stress you put it through."

As I sat alone on the marble dining table in my house, I asked myself if an overdose of this medication, mixed with other drugs for severe depression and anxiety, would be enough to push me over the edge. These thoughts of suicide had been getting stronger and stronger every day.

As a medical doctor, I knew how to dodge those questions when asked by the shrink, "Have you ever had any thoughts of harming yourself?" I knew that if I replied in affirmative to those tricky questions, then it would translate into a more severe diagnosis with more potent medications, and the term 'suicidal' would be added to my medical notes. That would be too stigmatizing, even though this was not the first time I had attempted to kill myself.

Just two months earlier, I had driven our red Toyota Corolla, commonly called an Uber-type because it was used by most Uber drivers due to its efficient fuel consumption, to the only artificial lake in Abuja where I parked my car, beside the Jabi Lake Bridge.

As Nigeria's capital city, Abuja does not have the luxury of having many bridges like the 11.8 km third mainland bridge in Lagos. It was the longest bridge in Africa until the 6th October Bridge in Cairo, Egypt, measuring 20.5 kilometers long, which took nearly 30 years to construct, was inaugurated in 1996. The third mainland bridge had also become infamous as the geographical location for many suicide attempts, with patrol teams available to stop people from jumping off the bridge and arresting them for failed attempts. It is quite absurd to be sent to prison for wanting to kill oneself.

I sat in my red Corolla, grappling with a weighty decision: should I jump off the bridge with the car key in hand or leave it behind in the ignition? The thought of leaving the keys behind nagged at me; a lucky thief could quickly drive away with my car. Anxiety coursed through me as I pondered, my heart racing as my thoughts spiraled out of control like the antics of Oga Sabinus—Emmanuel Chukwuemeka Ejekwu, the beloved Nigerian comedian known for his humorous skits and memes.

Just then, my phone buzzed: Osaigbovo Bello, an old friend from Federal Government College, Warri, called.

We had forged a close bond during high school in the historic city of Benin, Edo State, and he had only recently moved his family to Canada. We had not spoken in over a year, and now he was on the line, launching me into an endless conversation that stretched on for thirty minutes. You might call it a divine intervention, but as much as I appreciated the connection, I was growing weary and exhausted. I could sense the curious glances of passersby at my car parked precariously by the bridge. Reluctantly, I ended the call and drove back home. What a bugger!! I sighed.

Despite the interruption, I was determined not to let Gbovo, as I fondly called him, derail my plans. I had taken a cocktail of medications—at least ten tablets of Bisoprolol— hoping they would serve their intended purpose and slow down my racing heart. It was around 8 PM, and I resolved to go to bed, praying to wake up on the other side, but to my utmost surprise, I woke up with a start, glancing at the clock, only to find out that it was 11.45 PM, still the same day.

I was alive, but a sense of dread washed over me, and it felt as though I were leaving my body, my skin rolling back on itself. For the first time, I experienced a flicker of regret; I did not want to die. Was this an out-of-body experience? The last thing I remembered was walking toward the bathroom. When I regained consciousness, I found myself lying on the bed, and my neighbors gathered in our bedroom; yet, I had no recollection of inviting anyone over for a pajama party.

Later on that day, my wife narrated the incident that led to the gathering of the crowd; she said that she heard a loud thump by the bathroom door, a sound that marked my collapse to the floor. Since she could not lift me by herself, she quickly beckoned on the new maid to lend a helping hand. Right there, I imagined how bewildered the new maid must have been, wondering what kind of crazy house this was. Before then, she had recently seen prayer warriors visiting the house, and now this.

My wife said that when they attempted to lift me, I tried to protest, urging them to let me be, only for me to collapse again before being carried back to bed. She immediately and frantically called on our neighbors, hence their unexpected presence.

I felt a dual wave of embarrassment wash over me: First, I had survived yet another attempt, and second, I was acutely aware of what had happened but unable to voice it out to anyone. What kind of a person tries to end their life when they have a beautiful wife, a lovely son, and three cars parked outside their home? Apparently, that was 'Me'.

Depression is an equal-opportunity affliction that does not discriminate; unfortunately, it affects both the affluent and the impoverished, the old and the young, and it spares no one, not even those perceived as strong. It is impossible to pinpoint precisely when one becomes or the moment suicidal thoughts take root in one's mind. They creep in insidiously, tightening their grip until your entire thoughts and existence feel submerged beneath them.

While this should be the moment to seek help, your state of mind will definitely resist any form of assistance, concealing your pain even from doctors. The thoughts will become burdensome, growing heavier, suffocating you until escape through death seems like the only best option. Let's go back to my story.

We made a trip to the hospital in the wee hours of the morning despite my strong objections to my wife. At that point, my ability to make decisions for the family had dwindled; I was merely a spectator in my own life, informed of decisions made on my behalf.

Upon arriving at the hospital, we met with the young doctor who could not phantom and seemed baffled by my low blood pressure readings, considering the fact that I was a hypertensive patient. He was clearly irritated as he sent us home, instructing us to return for further evaluation the next day. Little did he know the impact an overdose of Bisoprolol could have on my blood pressure; still, I had no intention of enlightening him.

Sub-Chapter

"The reward for hard work is rest and not more hard work ... don't be fooled!"
- Andrew Etsetowaghan

As I continue to share my story, I sometimes wonder if it will one day resonate with someone who feels like they are the only one isolated on a similarly lonely road. When visiting a psychiatrist, you find yourself examining your lineage, questioning whether your struggles are genetic or simply unique to you. The "Why me?" dilemma looms large, and I have also started to undertake this task seriously. Let me share the details.

I was born via cesarean section in 1976 in Ibadan, leaving my mother with a longitudinal scar on her tummy that would ensure she is forever disqualified and never a contestant in any bikini contest. As the youngest of nine children in a monogamous household, I grew up in a complex family dynamic. Why? Because my mother had adopted four siblings from my father's extramarital adventures outside the confines of monogamy. This made it difficult to distinguish my step-siblings from my biological siblings until I was a teenager because my mom was a good stepmother, and I will always cherish her late memory. God bless her soul.

My educational journey took me from Corona School in Gbagada, Lagos, to Federal Government College Warri in what was then called Bendel State, now Delta State. I vividly remember traveling to my boarding school in Benin, then Bendel state, and returning to Benin in Edo state from my school, now in Delta state.

This happened in August 1991, during a political transition in Nigeria, when the military junta decided it was time to increase the number of states in Nigeria from 21 to 30 and eventually to 36 in 1996; at the time, I was in SS1 or what my son now calls 'Year 10'.

I studied medicine at the University of Benin for an initially proposed duration of six years. Still, I graduated nine years later due to repeated Academic Staff Union of Universities (ASSU) strikes.

My study duration in the College of Medicine was not uneventful as I passed through the university, and the university passed through me; perhaps my decision to join a confraternity in my very first year had something to do with this. However, it was a decision I regretted throughout my stay at the University as I could not phantom how a brotherhood would welcome you with a brutal beating with sticks in the name of initiation.

Right from the initiation night, I did everything that I could possibly do to put a clear distance between myself and the group, coupled with some divine reprieve coming in my 4th year with the disbandment of all 'cult groups'— that's a better name for these violent associations.

A few years later, in 2002, while completing my clinical internship at a military hospital in Lagos, I met a beautiful ebony-skin lady, Ehigocho, at the Doctors' lounge. She was a 3rd-year law student at the University of Jos at the time. This lady played a critical role in my survival and later became my wife in 2008 in a modest ceremony in Abuja.

It was during my compulsory one-year national youth service in Gombe State, in Northeast Nigeria, that I began to exhibit some troubling symptoms—perhaps the early signs of mental health issues. I had been biting my nails since childhood; maybe that was a possible indication of underlying anxiety that went unnoticed; in contrast, while studying for a Master's degree in Public Health in Leeds, United Kingdom, I seemed to navigate life successfully, graduating with distinctions and various awards.

Well, as I began to probe and check my mental health, a similar process medical students use in order to get clinical information from patients, I noticed a repeated pattern of sleep deprivation. As I grew in my career in the Public Health sphere, I saw another pattern of trying to be that superstar—the "star boy" everyone wanted to be in the organization showed up in me.

I remember telling a colleague of mine in my last job before I fell ill, "Old boy when I saw my salary, I felt like I would die working here"; ironically, the words almost came true. My wife often remarked to her friends, "My husband hardly sleeps; he is a workaholic." A co-worker once said, "If you email Dr. Andrew at 3:00am, he will respond by 3.02 am." That made me a night owl, giving me approximately one minute to read before replying.

Apart from that, music has always been a favorite pastime and passion of mine, perhaps inherited from my father, Mr. Emmanuel Etsetowaghan (Snr), who kept stacks of old vinyl records in our home and would play it through an interconnected network of wired speakers every Saturday. I enjoyed a wide range of genres—gospel, jazz, traditional music, and the increasingly popular Afro beats as long as they were of good quality.

I became an instant fan of Damini Ebunoluwa Ogulu, popularly known by the stage name Burna Boy when I was captivated by his fusion of Afro beats and hit songs such as *Ye, last-last, and Dangote*. Alhaji Aliko Dangote, Africa's richest man, inspired the latter's hit track "Dangote," the lyrics more than resonated with me as they captured a universal struggle.

"Dangote, Dangote Dangote still dey find money o
I no dey, I no dey
I no dey sleep on the money o
Who I be? Who I be? Wey make I no go find money o
I no dey send anybody o
Me, I dey hustle gan gan."

If Dangote, with all his wealth, was still restless at night, seeking more ways to create more wealth, then indeed, it was alright for me to sacrifice a little portion of my sleeping hours in pursuit of success; after all, I was not as wealthy as Alhaji Dangote—this was a self-hypnotic act, and I mentally gave myself a pat on the back.

But in January 2021, I fell ill seriously…

Here are a few questions that might help you discover any hidden or underlying issues with your mental health and possibly get answers that had seemed elusive.

Reflective Questions

1. Have you ever faced a situation that challenged your mental health?

2. What emotions did you experience during these challenges?

3. How did your relationship with yourself change after those experiences?

4. Did you find it challenging to open up about your struggles?

5. What support did you receive from others, and how did it impact you?

Chapter Two

THE DEADLY SPIRAL INTO BURNOUT

"You drown not by falling into the
water, but by staying submerged in it."
- Paulo Coelho

A year after my recovery, I had the opportunity to give
a talk on burnout, and the reactions of the audience
profoundly moved me. Many attendees shared stories
of loved ones who had experienced similar struggles, while a
few even recounted how burnout had tragically claimed the
life of a relative. I couldn't help but think that the COVID-19
pandemic, with its surge in virtual meetings and remote work,
had worsened the burnout crisis globally, particularly among
healthcare workers who found themselves on the frontlines,
their quality of life severely compromised.

During my presentation, I began by defining burnout to ensure everyone understood its core concept. An individual is said to experience burnout when they face a state of chronic physical and emotional exhaustion, detachment, and reduced efficiency related to their work or responsibilities. The World Health Organization (WHO) classifies burnout as an occupational phenomenon characterized by three primary dimensions:

1. **Emotional Exhaustion**: This involves feeling drained, overwhelmed, and emotionally depleted, leading to a sense of being unable to contribute further to one's work or responsibilities.

2. **Depersonalization:** Individuals may develop a cynical or detached attitude toward their work and the people they serve, leading to feelings of disconnection and a lack of empathy.

3. **Reduced Personal Accomplishment**: This manifests as a feeling of inadequacy and a decline in self-esteem, where individuals perceive themselves as ineffective in their roles and believe they are not achieving meaningful outcomes. To be diagnosed with burnout, these symptoms must persist for an extended period and significantly impact an individual's daily functioning, relationships, and overall quality of life.

It's important to note that burnout can stem from various factors, including excessive workload, lack of control, insufficient support, and imbalanced work-life dynamics. If someone recognizes these signs in themselves, then it is crucial to seek support and take actionable steps toward recovery.

But how did I find myself in the depths of burnout? It began when I was working on a grant proposal that had been delayed, and during that period, my sleeping hours were reduced significantly to zero; I would lie down in bed around 2 a.m. or 3 a.m., and somehow, I would find myself awake doing one thing or the other until morning.

I managed to function for some time, delegating tasks to my team, but my creativity and ability to think clearly vanished gradually; I recall struggling for hours on how to articulate my words for a PowerPoint presentation, stuck on the introductory slide without progressing a bit.

In my desperation, I reached out to a doctor friend for advice, and he offered a few suggestions, many of which I became accustomed to from various therapists in those coming months.

Determined to regain control of my life, I decided to tackle my sleeplessness all by myself by simply identifying a few rag-tag pharmaceutical shops at night and having a way around words; I obtained sleeping pills such as diazepam without a prescription. Miraculously, I found one pharmacy that sold Diazepam to me without asking for my doctor's Identity Card.

I started with 5mg of Diazepam, a famous sedative, and initially managed to get a weary two hours of sleep, which reduced to zero after a few nights. As a doctor, I knew the consequences of my actions, but I was desperate and no longer cared about the adverse effects.

I took another route by increasing my dosage to 10mg, then I was able to catch two hours of sleep, and that was all. Friends from my cycling club began to notice a few changes in my demeanor; Pastor Yemi even remarked, "Capo, you no longer laugh as usual."

Pastor Yemi is a fellow member of the Abuja Chaingang, a renowned mountain biking group I helped establish and later led as captain, earning me the nickname "Capo." As my lack of sleep deepened, I became paranoid; I began to overanalyze the simplest actions and words from my coworkers, magnifying minor mistakes until I felt the weight of the world pressing down on me. On the surface, I maintained an impeccable facade, but inside, I was a roller coaster of spiraling thoughts and emotions.

I had my life all planned out, yet it appeared as though I was the only one aware of what was happening to me, while others seemed to perceive me as being resistant to failure. In an attempt to reassure myself, I sought intimacy with my wife to test whether I was still the man I used to be by clinging to the hope that if I performed very well physically, that would be an indication that I was still okay.

Then, one evening, I faced every man's worst nightmare: erectile dysfunction. The realization struck me hard—my body began breaking down. My wife rushed me to the hospital, where I was admitted with severe hypertension, an enlarged heart, lipid disorders, and, of course, chronic insomnia. In my mind, if only I could sleep, then I would get the pieces of my life back together. The doctors seemed to agree at first and administered an intravenous sedative, expecting I would be knocked out for hours.

Nonetheless, an hour later, I woke up and felt my heart beating erratically, like a drummer who had drunk too much but refused to stop playing and resign to bed—It was so pronounced and audible that my wife could feel it from her side of the bed.

Once I got admitted, the alarm bells rang throughout my workplace, and my entire management team came to visit. They immediately insisted that my laptop and all work-related materials be taken away. My former boss, Mrs. Christy Laniyan, was a formidable leader, a real iron woman with a heart of gold, who had overcome various adversities to become one of the most respected Public Health personalities in Nigeria; she reminded my wife of how hardworking I was and what a great asset I was to her team. Christy Laniyan.

Although everyone seemed supportive, I found myself unable to sleep. My mobile phones were confiscated to ensure I could rest; however, rest did not come easy, and tranquility seemed elusive as I later understood that I had effectively mortgaged my sleep, which was no longer available on request. I spent two and half weeks in the hospital and was eventually discharged; I found my voice, but my spirit was still fragile.

Sub-Chapter

"Before something great happens, everything falls apart."
– Unknown

Before my two-week stay at the hospital, I had never been admitted for even a night in any hospital. Upon returning home, I did not feel any better as my hypertension had set in yet again, and I was now juggling a cocktail of daily medications.

My laptop had remained unopened for weeks—definitely an unprecedented Guinness World Record for me and on the second day after returning from the hospital, I made a regretful but fateful decision to open my Laptop to check in on work and get acquainted with what was happening at the office. I was the 'Big Boss' or the Technical Director, so I assumed and thought that the world revolved around me and it would surely stop if I did not go to work. I typed in my office password, and my mailbox opened and exploded with 3,457 unread messages.

Immediately, a sense of panic washed over me, and I felt a severe sharp pain in the left side of my chest. Memories of medical school flooded my brain— was this a heart attack? I called my wife to drive me to the hospital, and she jumped into her red Mercedes GLK 350 and drove off like a possessed woman.

As we got to the intersection of the main road, the pain worsened; desperate and frustrated, I told her to take a detour to church for my final blessing. The pain was excruciating and unbearable, and in a state of sheer panic, I asked my wife to place a call to our close family members and set her phone on hands-free mode as I needed to say my final goodbye and instruct them to look after my family.

With the clarity of hindsight, I realized I was experiencing a panic attack—something that would repeat itself in months to come. When we arrived at the hospital, my family members requested that I should be transferred immediately to another facility that was more responsive to their patient's needs. This decision turned out to be a critical step in the chain of events that led to a comedy of errors, misdiagnosis, and deepening mistrust.

On arrival at the 'new and bigger hospital,' it became evident that they did not have my medical records, thereby forcing me to undergo all the tests again. They were also pressured to perform and deliver results quickly and asked for urgent heart scans and ECG tests. Unfortunately, the regular Consultant Radiologist was away and unavailable that night, leaving a stand-in doctor to review my tests— the test results were inconclusive, and I was admitted once again.

It was an awful night; my wife and son were broken and totally disorganized, and I yet could not sleep. The following day, I had many visitors and family members, but the hospital's lack of understanding and regard for visiting hours only heightened my anxiety. This was meant to be a show of love; instead, it became overwhelming.

During the doctor's ward rounds, the sudden chest pain returned, once again resembling a heart attack, prompting them to administer medication for relief. I could hear the doctors speaking in our usual jargon, including the stand-in doctor from the previous night, who recommended another expensive test at a different hospital. Notably, the human heart releases certain substances under stress; however, we did not receive the test result then, so they couldn't decipher what was happening to me.

On hearing the Doctor's recommendation, I was quickly whisked away in an ambulance to a third hospital managed by a Turkish team. There, I was scheduled to have a minor surgery procedure involving the insertion of a rubber tube with a camera passed from my thigh to my heart through a central vein. It sounded terrifying, and I found myself merely observing as Ehi(my wife) and relatives made all the arrangements.

The procedure went pretty fast after a deposit of $2000 was made. They discovered that my heart was very normal for a man in his mid-forties; however, I was getting more irritated, and my frustration mounted as I was still unable to sleep. The foreign doctor then mentioned quietly to my wife the need to see a psychiatrist.

I later understood that the doctor who referred me for the procedure received a percentage of money for my referral. I was met with a different reception upon going to the hospital that I had been referred to. The doctors began to avoid my room during their rounds even though I was also a doctor; this was my first encounter with the stigma associated with perceived mental illness.

By the second week, I was informed I would see a behavioral physician; I guess this was a fancy name for a psychiatrist, designed to minimize the stigmatization effect for both the doctors and their patients. This was to be my first encounter with a shrink, and although she was Muslim, she was able to probe through my defenses, prescribing new drugs that were not covered by my health insurance—those drugs, she assured me, would help me sleep.

I bought the story, and we had our networks search and scour the entire Lagos until we found them. Unfortunately, they only managed to give me two hours of sleep, leaving me feeling exhausted each time I woke up. Ugh! I hated my life.

Soon, it became apparent that the hospital understood that they were not doing much for me other than racking up a massive bill for my organization, which paid for my health insurance. I later realized that mental health illness was so stigmatized to the extent that the behavioral physician had to use another ailment to get her bills paid. My diagnosis eventually was presented as a mixed anxiety-affective disorder; in a lay-person's terms, I was gradually spiraling into depression and anxiety.

Once again, I had to face the daunting task of returning home, still not sleeping, and taking medications for my anxiety and mild depression. Yet, the truth was that my depression was anything but mild. I knew what answers to give to distract the doctor, but the doctor was also good at probing deeper because she would ask, in a hundred different ways, if I had any suicidal thoughts. As usual, I would respond with a resounding "No" each time she asked, even though the answer began to shift toward "Yes" in the back of my mind for some of the questions.

Sub-Chapter

"It is not enough to be compassionate – you must act."
- The Dalai Lama

I would not have described myself as religious or spiritual during that tumultuous period. Still, I have always known there was a greater being, and I have always had a strong intuitive spirit— Some people describe this as divine providence. However, during the lockdown, an overwhelming urge compelled me to drive to a local church and donate money to the Parish priest. I felt this deep burden in my heart and did this several times throughout the lockdown period.

During one of my panic attacks, I asked my wife to reach out to the church for prayers; the Parish Priest I had supported was unavailable, but he sent his assistant, who coincidentally shared my first name. When he entered my hospital room, his piercing gaze scanned the space, and I couldn't help but recall scenes from "*The Exorcist*," wondering if my head might spin through 360 degrees.

We went through the regular prayers, holy communion, and the "give your life to Christ" routine. It seemed a bit distant at first as I was down and in a dark place, willing to do any prayer that might help me get better; it did not feel real, in fact, I felt guilty for playing along. Nevertheless, over the few months of the following year, I became quite close to Rev Father Andrew Sule, and we would spend quite some time together every day; I began to see the humanity in his words and shared wisdom.

Later on, I learned from him that he had suffered burnout at an outstation, and from the moment he laid eyes on me in the hospital, he recognized the pain that my eyes could not conceal. I wanted a quick solution and rejected the notion that it could take me at least a year or more to recover.

That notion felt absurd to him because I just needed to sleep, and I would be better, and everything would fall into place. He was right: Rome was not built in a day, but was it really destroyed in one? Take a few minutes to self-reflect while answering these questions.

Reflections

1. How do you recognize the early signs of burnout or stress in yourself?

2. What steps can you take to address them before they escalate?

3. How did your relationship with loved ones change after your experience?

3

Chapter Three

MORE THAN MEETS THE EYE

"Don't depend too much on anyone in this
world because even your own shadow leaves
you when you are in darkness."
- Ibn Taymiyyah

I was discharged from the hospital once again, making it three months since the whole ordeal began, yet no solution was in sight. Before I fell ill, I had been working for an international non-profit or Non-governmental organization renowned for having one of the best human resources departments; nonetheless, as I faced the reality of my situation, I felt a pressing need to return to work.

Even though my boss generously offered me a month or as long as I needed, I sensed the bitter truth behind those comforting words he provided. Guilt gnawed at me as I collected a paycheck while contributing little or nothing to the organization's progress. So, after a month of this internal struggle, I made one of the worst decisions of my life: Returning to work without getting better and before I was truly ready.

On resuming work, I was greeted with a barrage of emails from colleagues expressing gratitude to God for my healthy comeback. Were these people nuts and out of touch with reality? I was barely managing two hours of sleep each night, thanks to a cocktail of medications that would leave me in a fog all day. Each time I was about to take my medications, I would be reminded of my late mother, who had a jar filled with pills for almost everything—both necessary and unnecessary illnesses.

She had these expensive multivitamins sent by my brother in the United Kingdom, which she would mix with other vitamins from some local shops in Nigeria. Each visit to her was a challenge as I would always have a hard time sifting through her myriad of medications. The only difference now was that I hadn't yet resorted to the various balms for arthritis that had given her room a distinct, lingering scent. She passed away in 2015 before any of these began else; it would have probably killed her to see her son suffer as I did.

Back at the office, I quickly realized that my memory was a bit altered as I had difficulty remembering some things— it became short-term, which meant that I struggled to remember the names of individuals I had met the previous day. This was shocking, considering that I had been one of the top graduates from the University of Leeds' Master of Public Health program. What was happening to me? Fortunately, our meetings remained virtual due to ongoing social distancing measures, allowing me to navigate my responsibilities successfully —until the breaking point arrived.

Two weeks after returning to work, I was asked to provide insights on a critical issue as the program's technical director. I blanked out entirely and was caught in an unsettling silence that filled the virtual room. Gratefully, someone suggested that I might be experiencing problems with my internet connection, and the meeting continued; still, I felt utterly humiliated. Afterward, I called my boss and explained to her what happened. Christy Laniyan, a boisterous, family-oriented leader, promptly contacted my wife to pick me up from the office.

Despite being paid my remuneration, I had exhausted all possible excuses for leave and was only receiving my basic salary, excluding allowances; with time, I began to drift into the dark abyss known as depression. Also, I had stopped taking or making phone calls of any sort, and I just wanted to be left alone and withdraw into a shell, not caring about my welfare or personal hygiene. I would only have my bath at 5 P.m. when I heard my wife return from work. The reality hit me: My sense of self-worth had vanished, and it was clear I was no longer the breadwinner or the decision-maker in our home anymore.

I recalled my medical school professor listing out the cardinal symptoms of depression: sadness, anxiety, hopelessness, worthlessness, and anhedonia. Anhedonia is a unique symptom where a person finds it impossible to find joy or enjoy any activity. I felt all this and more, but my greatest fear was losing my job.

I had stopped watching television and wanted it put off permanently; similarly, my laptop had gathered dust, running so slowly that it needed multiple software updates; my wife had then begun taking on chores that were typically mine previously. However, a good side to all these was that my erectile dysfunction had improved, and my sex drive had increased—this was something I later learned was a side effect of a specific medication.

My once-vibrant social network dwindled to just a handful of friends—three or four who still cared and were thoughtful enough to check in on me. It was at that period that I realized that the easiest way to turn people away was simply not to return their calls; a few would try again, but most of them would take one missed or unreturned call as a sign to retreat, only reaching out if they had something to gain. This principle rings true, as I have witnessed how deserted the homes of certain politicians become after they leave their political offices.

Ope Abiodore, my roommate and adopted brother from Leeds University, was one of the few who stood by me. We were both medical doctors, but I was much older and had often pushed him to do better in our studies and on most issues then. Ope is laid back but extremely intelligent and cerebral. I remembered how he had come to me to help him with a Health Economics assignment and ended up scoring the highest in the class when our results came out; meanwhile, I barely had a passing grade of 60.

For some time, Ope had been bugging me to grant him an opportunity to visit me, but I declined, so he eventually stopped asking, understanding that I would refuse. Instead, for over six months, he dedicated his weekends to making the long hours of drive to my home in Abuja just to check up on someone who did not want to see or receive anyone.

Sub-Chapter

"To share your weakness is to make yourself vulnerable; to make yourself vulnerable is to show your strength"
- Criss Jami.

Throughout my struggles, both my family and my wife's family had been unwavering in their support; yet, an unspoken campaign began to emerge, aiming to explore alternative solutions to my plight.

In Africa, there often exists a tendency to externalize our challenges, especially when they remain persistent. I believe the continent of Africa is likely to have the highest numbers of churches, Pastors, traditional healers, and witch doctors, or Babalawos, in the world; Nigeria, in particular, is probably home to some of the largest churches globally, both in size and congregation.

A family member soon suggested visiting one of the then 'trendy Men of God' to seek possible healing during his weekly service; obviously, I was open and receptive to any potential solution in my state of vulnerability. We arrived at the church early, around 6 a.m., to secure decent seats near the front row, even though the actual deliverance service wouldn't commence until the next three hours.

The atmosphere was electrifying, filled with vibrant singing and dancing as the congregation prepared for the main event. As the service unfolded, the auditorium became very similar to a scene from a 1980s horror movie, with people falling on the ground and rolling uncontrollably in displays of emotion.

While I may not be in a position to question the authenticity of the miracles being performed, the testimonies shared were abundant. I held onto the infallible hope that I, too, might experience mine, even as the preacher passed by me multiple times without saying a word. Ultimately, we returned home that day without the so much anticipated healing we had sought.

We later sought another Man of God, who even visited us at home for a personal deliverance service. We had to provide funds for his transportation to-and-fro when it appeared that his usual two-hour visit yielded little relief. However, when he requested further visits, we politely declined, realizing the futility of the situation.

Five months into my illness, I was still unable to pinpoint the source of my affliction or what was wrong with me despite having worked as a medical doctor for over 20 years, as I could only articulate my symptoms. I still had persistent poor sleep and was depressed with intermittent panic attacks, which rendered me largely non-functional.

Our families unanimously decided that a total change of environment and a medical assessment outside the country might help provide clarity. As a result, my wife, son, and I traveled to the UK when the COVID-19 pandemic struck. The journey was possibly the most challenging, if not the worst, trip of my life as it was compounded by the discomfort of nasal swabs for COVID testing and a mandatory ten-day quarantine at my brother's house in the United Kingdom.

We stayed with my immediate elder brother, his wife, and their two adult children in their compact four-bedroom "London" house. It still amazes me how conservative British homes can be regarding the number of bathrooms to have in a family house because it's likely that the culture of queuing up to take turns to bath may have started in these British homes.

My brother, Emmanuel "Tunde" Etsetowaghan (Jnr), was the perfect host, though I sensed my nephew and niece were quite unsure and puzzled by the unexpected visit of their uncle and his entire family. I remember Tunde asking me, "Why don't you laugh anymore?"

The illness had begun to take a significant physical and emotional toll on my wife and son because even though I was physically present with them, I felt emotionally detached. My son had missed his term exams and was growing resentful toward me; he had seen his hero change into someone no one could recognize at the time, and his grades had also taken a nosedive; meanwhile, my wife was doing all she could to fill the void I had left.

The private healthcare assessment by the health providers in the UK was irrelevant, as I observed junior doctors simply recommended extensive baseline tests, seemingly to inflate the bills. I did, however, have a virtual consultation with a psychiatrist connected to my brother's church, who provided counsel and prayer. We returned to Nigeria after a whole month in the UK, with a slight improvement in my condition, and by then, eight months had passed since I had last functioned normally or worked.

I made a final attempt to return to work, but it was futile as I had lost the zeal to work, and my memory was faltering and not as good as it used to be. I struggled to go back to the office, and even when I did, I found myself drifting into the world of dark thoughts as there were some days I would drive to work but park a few blocks away from the office, lost in contemplation and drowning myself in thoughts. I was fighting many internal demons, and it was on one of those fateful days that I found myself parked on the side of the bridge in my Corolla, contemplating to end it all.

Having been out of a job for over nine months, I still held a significant management position in my organization, and the meeting I had dreaded finally arrived. I vividly remember Audu Amushe, the head of HR, tearfully discussing the mutual agreement for my resignation; fortunately, the organization provided additional financial support through our group health insurance policy to enable me to augment my upkeep and expenses in the subsequent months. I hold no grudges against them; in fact, I returned to the office a year later to talk about burnout after my recovery.

I ran into Dr Bridget Nwagbara at the HR desk during my final exit documentation at the office. I had met Bridget just once before that day, as most of our management meetings were done virtually. I had stood behind her in a queue to get our COVID jab in the office but exchanged pleasantries only briefly. She told me she heard that I was ill and apparently had suffered a similar illness and promised to visit my wife and me at home, to which she later called to get directions to my house.

Now, let's take some time to ponder these questions; perhaps they might change your perspective about seeking help, repairing, or strengthening the relationship ties with your loved ones.

Reflections

1. What have you learned about the value of life and the importance of seeking help?

2. What lessons have you learned about the importance of seeking professional help?

3. Have you ever acted in a way that affected your loved ones?

4. What have you learned about the importance of considering the impact of your actions on others?

5. How can you work to repair any damage caused by your past actions?

4

Chapter Four

MEETING BRIDGET NWAGBARA

"My recovery must come first so that everything
I love in life doesn't have to come last."
– Unknown

"How I (Bridget) got involved…"

It was in the month of April 2021; while waiting in line for the first dose of the COVID-19 vaccine, I bumped into Andrew Etsetowaghan, who was ahead of me in the queue. We shared a few jokes about the scientific controversies surrounding the vaccine and concluded that we had nothing to lose by taking it. After that day, I didn't know that it would take a few months before I saw him again, but it would be under a completely different circumstance.

Bridget's Story…

I had just become a mother and was excited about the prospects of exclusive breastfeeding as I knew the benefits it offered for both the mother and the baby. From my previous experience, I enjoyed how it helped me shed pregnancy weight with minimal effort, and I wanted to experience it again; nevertheless, no two babies behave in the same way because I realized that my healthy and energetic baby boy had a huge appetite.

That made me breastfeed him on demand, even though I was eating, making me feel as light as a feather. At that time, I could drink up to three liters of water at a time and spend my day making it revolve around eating, drinking, breastfeeding, and napping.

Eight weeks into this carefully managed routine, I started to feel very tired. I also noticed that I had stopped going out as often as I did, suffered from more headaches than usual, and my sleep was suffering, too; this was particularly the most challenging part for me because I have always loved my sleep. Yet, I was also losing weight, and as my maternity leave was coming to an end, that made me grow increasingly concerned about my health.

Seeking medical help seemed like the right step; however, different doctors offered different opinions on my fatigue and weight loss, which only added to my already jumbled state of confusion. Amid this uncertainty and confusion, a close friend recommended Dr. Abah.

I was fortunate to meet Dr. Abah, who looked me straight in the face and said, "Childbirth and breastfeeding can be incredibly stressful. Do you understand the changes that your body has gone through? Do you understand the impact of stress on your health? What diagnosis are you looking for? You are severely stressed! You need to focus on recovery and rest".

I felt he was oversimplifying a grave issue. I also expressed my worries to him about being too exhausted and wanting to return to work once my maternity leave ended. "How can I go back to work in this state?" I needed clarification. Then he asked, "Do you need to go to work? What exactly is your priority? You are stressed and need to rest".

My husband, who I suspected was on a mission to get me off work, agreed with him and told him that I did not have to go back to work; just like that, my fate was sealed, and I could not resume work after three months of maternity leave—as an independent consultant, no work meant no earnings.

Dr Abah looked at me and said, "What exactly is so important about work besides making money? That is what we need to address in order to help you heal." All he did was advise me to go home and reflect on my relationship with work. For me, work has never been just about earning an income; it is more about something I cannot pinpoint today, and it is complex. Yes, I admit that it is not solely about lending my head, heart, and hands to solving complex public health problems.

Throughout my maternity leave, I would hang out with friends, laughing and enjoying their company, without telling them about my struggles and what I was going through. They had no idea of my fatigue, and I guess that is why they cheered me on about the weight loss and relaxed look. Still, they had no idea what reality was at home. Why did I create this charade about my well-being? Why didn't I decline some of the meetings I attended even while on maternity leave? You are about to find out.

During my maternity leave, I guided a work colleague through the analysis of her data for her Master's thesis program. She reached out in distress, explaining that without my help in completing the thesis, she wouldn't be able to graduate, hence why she needed my help; so, without a sense of self-preservation, despite the sleep deprivation and headaches, I offered to help her.

This meant reviewing her methodology, pointing out the errors, and then guiding her to apply the correct codes in the data analysis software to get the correct answers. I did this to the chagrin of my husband and loved ones, who knew what I was going through then. This experience highlighted my unhealthy relationship with work, but I could have said no, and our relationship would have remained unchanged.

Remember, at that time, I was still breastfeeding exclusively, and even when my family did everything in their power to discourage me from what they felt was self-sacrifice, I pressed on. I was committed to breastfeeding until the recommended six months.

My husband, who had a strong background in trauma and brain health, urged me to reflect on the underlying causes of my fatigue and sleep deprivation. He told me I needed to say goodbye to work, emphasizing that I had to choose between my well-being and my job, and also warned that I risked prolonged suffering and healing if I didn't make a change.

Dr. Abah echoed the sentiments and cautioned me that I could continue the charade and end up with a lifetime of fatigue and headaches. He explained that while medications might help me function properly, they wouldn't provide true healing—That thought was scary, and I longed for the fatigue to dissipate and to return to my active lifestyle.

Notably, I was a recreational runner before my maternity leave, jogging 2.5 kilometers thrice a week. So, after eight weeks of postpartum, I returned to morning walks and jogged for four months. However, during his time, I found myself becoming a couch potato, and staying like one for the rest of my life wasn't something I wanted. It was a fate that I was determined to avoid—I just had to do something.

I took my husband's advice and decided to quit work entirely. We went to a bookshop to get books that I could read during my time off work. Dr. Abah recommended and encouraged me to resume walking no matter how tired I felt, and I did exactly that. My pace was painfully slow at first, but I kept going, and after each hour-long walk, I would come home, hydrate, eat, and then sleep. To my surprise, I began to sleep soundly, and the sleep was highly refreshing, and I started compensating for the sleep deprivation at night.

Without the pressure of work hanging over me, I continued this routine until my strength gradually returned; I realized that I was then able to sit through the day without napping for long periods, and my nights became more restful as I started sleeping at night, and the headaches gradually faded.

In addition to physical activity, Dr. Abah recommended meditation, telling me to try my best to focus on something other than reading. It was very difficult at first, if not impossible, as I either slept off or my thoughts ran amok; despite everything that happened, he still encouraged me to keep trying to focus on gazing at even a door knob for one minute, and so, I started staring at the doorknob in front of my couch for a minute. Gradually, a minute became five minutes until I could do the meditation sessions successfully. I observed that the headaches faded completely while I focused on the doorknob, and this made me dive deeper into meditation. Eventually, I discovered Vipassana meditation, which I practice today.

The fatigue and the headaches were the most significant symptoms that I had, and that combination nearly spiraled me out of control. As soon as I was able to rein them in, I gradually returned to the person I knew before— A combination of physical activity and meditation got me back on my feet.

By that time, I had disappeared from the formal work scene; as you know, Public Health is a career that revolves around attending meetings, and a person can't be gone without being noticed as people would ask questions and expect explanations to be offered. Extended maternity leave is not a norm in my field, and soon enough, work came calling, but this time, my perspective shifted because my well-being took precedence. I was determined to prioritize it above all else.

Sub-Chapter

"We don't meet people in life by mere chance; They are meant to cross our Paths for a reason."

It was a tense and challenging year for the Global Fund Project, which Andrew managed as the Technical Director. Beyond the hurdles posed by COVID-19, they were also operating in very tense terrain. Anambra State, one of the Global Fund's priority states, had an upcoming election later in that year. It was also the epicenter of the rising tensions from the secessionist group, Indigenous People of Biafra (IPOB).

The Senior Management Meetings were where we brainstormed strategies to prepare for and mitigate the impact of these challenges on project implementation. Coupled with the physical distancing, which meant that we had to rely on the Microsoft Teams application for communication, we, unfortunately, experienced poor internet connectivity, which prevented us from using videos often, making virtual gatherings feel impersonal and detached—imagine a meeting with over 20 participants where you can't see anybody's face!

At that time, I doubted if those circumstances would allow us to offer adequate social and emotional support to the Global Fund Project during those challenging times. Yet, there was always one person who managed to lighten up the mood and get everyone laughing through his sense of humor: Andrew Etsetowaghan.

But then the jokes and laughter stopped coming, and I started asking questions until I was told that Andrew was very ill. Respecting his privacy and confidentiality, no one disclosed the nature of his condition; nevertheless, I kept asking about him because his jokes were very dear to me and had become a vital part of our team dynamics.

I had the opposite of Andrew's personality, which means that I believed that serious situations required a serious approach; to me, someone who could inject humor into grave issues while still delivering results was nothing short of magical– I missed that magic and was determined to find it again. With that determination, I reached out to a mutual close friend to learn more about what exactly was wrong with Andrew and his current situation, and that was the moment I was informed of multiple medical problems that did not seem to add up.

However, after getting the information, I gave it an afterthought, and it suddenly clicked, creating a eureka moment. I suggested to our mutual friend that I suspected Andrew was experiencing burnout, and she said, "AHA!" We both recognized and understood how exhaustion could lead to cardiovascular, metabolic, and psychological problems, and both of us knew that we had to share this perspective on his medical problems with him. So, we decided to pay him a home visit; however, that same afternoon, I unexpectedly bumped into him as he came to clear his desk—he had resigned.

I summoned the courage, went up to him, introduced myself, and asked if he recalled our conversation during the COVID-19 vaccination exercise. He laughed and said, "I know you very well." Then I told him that I would call him to fix a visit to his home as I had something important to discuss with him.

On getting home, I shared Andrew's experience with my husband, expressing my firm belief that my colleague was simply passing through extreme exhaustion; I felt that without the right intervention, Andrew would continue to believe he had a severe medical problem.

My husband agreed to accompany me on our visit, so we visited Andrew and his lovely wife that Sunday evening. There, we shared our experience with Dr. Abah, and I told him that I suspected he had a burnout. Like the natural comedian he is, he nearly fell off his seat laughing and said that I must be joking with him. How could I dare to simplify all he has been through to something as simple as a burnout?

His wife, nevertheless, had a different opinion because she described her husband as a workaholic who rarely slept or ate well. His regular physical activity of mountain biking had been abandoned for almost a year, leaving him just plain exhausted without any clear reason. She believed they had nothing to lose by exploring new avenues for healing. I don't know what she expected to hear, but she was surprised when I suggested that his healing process could involve morning bikes and getting some much-needed sleep in the morning.

I knew Andrew would not take my advice unless I explained the scientific basis of burnout and the recommendations I was making; therefore, to make it more real, I embarked on a deep dive into brain chemistry with him, and we went through the functions of each neurotransmitter.

It was an intensive four-hour visit where I explained how chronic stress can disrupt the release and function of these neurotransmitters and how they interact with other organs to manifest worrisome symptoms. There can be an imbalance in critical neurotransmitters such as serotonin, dopamine, and norepinephrine, and this imbalance can affect mood, motivation, and overall mental health.

Also, when you experience stress, your body releases stress hormones like cortisol; a high cortisol level over a long period can interfere with the normal functioning of neurotransmitters, which are the chemicals that transmit signals in the brain. Overall, chronic stress disrupts the delicate balance and function of neurotransmitters, which can lead to problems like anxiety, depression, and other mental health issues.

In the end, Andrew and his wife agreed to try morning cycling, saying that, after all, he was currently out of work and had nothing to lose. Although it wasn't an easy journey, he persevered. One day, we received a call that he had attended a wedding; then, the moment we had all been waiting for finally arrived—Andrew was ready to return to work.

After the excitement subsided, he told me he couldn't believe how much morning cycling had revitalized him, and he vowed to become an ambassador for burnout prevention— I'm pleased to say that he has stayed true to his word. Now, this is no longer about Andrew but YOU. Take some time to reflect deeply on the questions below.

Reflections

1. Did you experience any burnout during the COVID-19 pandemic?

2. What were the warning signs of burnout that you experienced, and how did you initially respond to them?

3. Who do you turn to for support when you feel overwhelmed, and how can you strengthen these relationships?

4. What self-care strategies (like exercise, meditation, or volunteering) do you currently practice?

5. Which new ones will you love to try?

Chapter Five

MENTAL HEALTH SERVICES IN NIGERIA AND THE ROLE OF THE CHURCH

Anyone living in Nigeria who says they don't
need a psychiatrist needs a Psychiatrist.

The above interesting but thought-provoking statement, originally penned by Kathy Lette about life in Los Angeles, resonates deeply when I adapt it to the Nigerian context.

My own experiences with psychiatrists—both before and after my illness-have been a mixed bag. I have encountered the Good and the Ugly, but thankfully not the bad, as I remember the classic 1966 western epic, "The Good, the Bad and the Ugly," starring Clint Eastwood.

One psychiatrist, in particular, left a lasting impression on me with his humility and sensitivity during my time in the abyss. First of all, we met in a very tranquil and serene location, far from the sterile, often intimidating atmosphere of a conventional hospital.

This was very reassuring and relaxing, as the fear of being "locked up" was eliminated, and you would not have the distinct oppressive smell of disinfectants and death that often accompany government hospitals. I'm convinced that this unconventional yet comforting approach needs further review to assess its potential benefits.

Dr. Sam Abah, a consultant Neuropsychiatrist with a difference, based in Abuja, stands out as one of my favorite people in the field. I spoke with him recently about the pressing need to have a book aimed at helping people going through various mental challenges, and he graciously agreed to share his insights, which are below.

In Nigeria and Africa at large, our view on mental health issues is largely shaped and influenced. Too often, mental health conditions are linked with spiritism or attributed to evil spirits and forces, overshadowing orthodox medical perspectives. Consequently, mental health services in Nigeria remain rudimentary, as insufficient attention has been directed toward this critical area of health care. Let's see how mental health treatment is being negatively influenced.

1. Cultural Beliefs and Stigma:

The association of mental health conditions with witchcraft or evil spirits is deeply ingrained in many societies and serves as a significant root of stigmatization, discrimination, and social isolation. This cultural belief often leads to the marginalization of individuals experiencing mental health issues, as they are perceived not only as suffering from an illness but also as being under the influence of malevolent forces.

The prevalence of derogatory terms such as "crazy," "mad," or the colloquial "Kolo mental" as the slang for mental health issues perpetuates the stigma, causing families to conceal any member of their family perceived to have a mental illness. Consequently, many individuals hesitate to seek help or openly discuss their mental health struggles, fearing rejection or ostracism.

In my experience consulting in the clinic, I have frequently encountered patients brought to the mental health clinic who express reluctance to engage with mental health services due to these misconceptions. On several occasions, patients have confronted me with statements like "Are you a psychiatrist? I don't want to see a psychiatrist; I am not mad."

This reflects a deeply rooted cultural misunderstanding that associates psychiatry solely with the treatment of severe mental illness, often overlooking the fact that mental health care encompasses a wide range of conditions, including anxiety, depression, and stress-related disorders.

The stigma surrounding mental health is not only detrimental to individuals but also hinders overall community well-being. Families often feel compelled to hide their loved ones' struggles, which can exacerbate feelings of loneliness and despair. This secrecy prevents open discussions about mental health, depriving communities of the opportunity to educate themselves about the importance of mental wellness and available resources.

2. Ignorance of Available Help and Treatments:

A significant number of Nigerians are not aware that they can seek help and treatments for the mental health problems confronting them by consulting mental health professionals. Consequently, many resort to faith-based healers or traditional remedies; this ignorance leads to delayed or inadequate care, resulting in increased morbidity and mortality from mental health illness.

My experiences with mental health patients have revealed that in most cases before the patient comes to the hospital, they must have sought help either from churches, mosques, or traditional healers; the hospital is seen as the last resort when others fail, and most people are skeptical about giving it a try, but by the time they arrive, skepticism often clouds their expectations.

3. Lack of Adequate Mental Health Professionals and Services:

The scarcity of mental health professionals—psychiatrists, mental health nurses, psychologists, and counselors—along with a limited number of specialized mental health hospitals and clinics, worsens the ongoing mental health crisis. This shortage is particularly pronounced in underserved regions, where the demand for mental health services far outstrips the available supply.

According to the World Health Organization, many countries have fewer than one psychiatrist per 100,000 people, highlighting a critical gap in mental health care resources. Furthermore, the few available services are concentrated in urban areas, making it highly challenging for individuals in rural communities to access the care they need.

In rural settings, transportation barriers, stigma surrounding mental health, and lack of awareness about available services can deter individuals from seeking help. Telehealth options have emerged as a potential solution to bridge this gap, but many rural areas still lack reliable internet access, limiting the effectiveness of such services.

Additionally, the workforce shortage is compounded by high rates of burnout among mental health professionals, often due to overwhelming caseloads and insufficient support. This situation is further aggravated by the rising prevalence of mental health issues, including anxiety, depression, and substance use disorders, which have surged in the wake of the COVID-19 pandemic.

4. Inadequate Funding and Lack of Political Will:

The disparity between available healthcare services and the need for mental health services in Nigeria is palpable as there is limited access to available and affordable health services, with many paying health expenses out-of-pocket.

Mental health services in Nigeria receive less funding and resources compared to other healthcare sectors. Nigeria's health sector and health services are mainly financed through the public sector financed through taxes, the private sector financed through voluntary insurance schemes, and the social security sector financed through obligatory insurance schemes for only people in the formal sector.

The mental health budget, funded mainly through the central government health budget, is about 3.3–4%, with over 90% going to the few neuropsychiatric hospitals available in Nigeria. This shortage of resources affects the availability and quality of mental health services; despite the rising cases of mental health issues in society, most healthcare facilities offer little or just skeletal mental health services due to insufficient funding to establish a functional mental health service delivery unit.

For example, when my health center wanted to build a block for mental health, it took several years of advocacy, presenting the proposal and budget to the National Assembly before it was approved, and even now, it has taken over three years. Completion remains stalled due to financial constraints.

In order to address these challenges, it is necessary to promote mental health services and increase mental health literacy via electronic media, newspapers, and social media. Mental health professionals, private organizations, and digital health companies, as part of their corporate social responsibility (CSR), can provide accessible and available digital platforms to give counseling, guidance on mental health issues, and a referral system to mental health care.

There is a need for the National Orientation Agency (NOA) to collaborate with the Federal Ministry of Health (FMOH) to create more strategic communication and coordinate public education and awareness campaigns on mental health and mental disorders, especially within educational institutions, communities, and rural areas. This will go a long way to reduce the stigma associated with mental illness.

Furthermore, incorporating culturally sensitive practices into mental health care can make services more accessible and acceptable to those who might otherwise avoid them. By engaging with community leaders, religious organizations, and local influencers, mental health professionals can better address the unique beliefs and values of different populations, paving the way for a more compassionate and inclusive approach to mental health care.

Primary health care is usually the first point of care and contact within the healthcare system. In many countries around the world, treatment, integration, and provision of mental health care through the primary health system have been practiced for a very long time. Integrating and providing mental health care and treatment through primary health care will enhance access, affordability, and cost-effectiveness. This can also serve as a site for rural postings for psychiatric residents training and practicing primary care physicians and nurses.

There is a need for a reform of the outdated existing laws and formulation of new policies that will see to the establishment of a commission for mental health with a mission to protect and support persons with mental health needs in Nigeria. Policymakers must also prioritize mental health in public health discussions and allocate funding to improve mental health infrastructure, ensuring that everyone has access to the care they need regardless of their geographic location.

In summary, challenging the stigma associated with mental health conditions is crucial for fostering a supportive environment where individuals feel safe to seek help. Through education, community engagement, and culturally informed practices, we can work toward breaking down barriers and promoting a more positive perception of mental health and well-being.

Role of the Church

"All it takes is a beautiful fake smile to hide an injured soul, and they will never know how broken you truly are."
- Robin Williams

Eighteen months after my recovery, I found myself captivated by a film titled *The Pope's Exorcist*, starring Russell Crowe, during my travels to Australia for a conference. The movie explores the life of Father Gabriele Amorth, the chief exorcist for the Vatican, who battles Satan and the demons that possess the innocent. The film paints a detailed portrait of a priest who performed over 100,000 exorcisms throughout his lifetime.

A particularly thought-provoking dialogue occurs between Father Amorth, Cardinal Sullivan, and Bishop Lumumba, where they discuss the issues of exorcisms.

Bishop Lumumba: "Cardinal Sullivan, in my observation, 98% of cases assigned to Father Amorth are recommended by him to Doctors and Psychiatrists."

Cardinal Sullivan: "And the other 2%?"

Father Amorth: (in Russel Crowe's voice) "Ah, the other 2%. This is something that has confounded all science and medicine for a very long time. I call it evil."

During my own illness, I noticed a contrasting trend in modern-day Pentecostalism, where over 98% or more of mental illnesses were attributed to some evil or demonic forces, with only 0-2% being ascribed to idiosyncratic causes. I recall instances from the early 2000s when HIV patients discontinued their medications after reportedly being "cured" at a church revival. This raises an important question about the profound influence of religion, often described as the opium of the masses.

In the depths of my illness, I encountered several religious figures who claimed to be able to perform instant miracles. In moments of vulnerability, we often seek solutions in every possible direction. While I do not doubt the existence of miracles, I also believe that our lord Jesus Christ did not operate as a magician.

From my limited understanding of the Holy Book, I often wondered why some miracles did not just happen with a simple wave of the hand. Why didn't He turn the water into wine in their glasses or instruct the 5000 to simply reach into their pockets for bread and fish?

Father Andrew Sule VC, a priest who supported me during my ailment, graciously shared his insights on the Church's role in addressing mental health. His perspective helped me navigate the complexities of faith, healing, and the interplay between spiritual beliefs and medical understanding.

The Catholic Church and Mental Health: A Perspective by Father Andrew Sule

Jesus said: *"The king will say to those on his right, 'Come, blessed of my Father! Take possession of the kingdom prepared for you from the beginning of the world. For I was hungry, and you fed me. I was thirsty, and you gave me something to drink. I was a stranger, and you welcomed me into your home. I was sick, and you visited me. I was in prison, and you came to see me."* – Matthew 25:34-36.

Upon examining this profound passage from the bible, a question comes to mind: Who truly comprehends the bitter experiences of hunger and thirst? Who feels like a stranger stripped of human dignity and pride? Who simultaneously feels sick and imprisoned within themselves? The answer points to anyone who has mental illness in any form.

As St. John Paul II stated in 1996, *"Whoever suffers from mental illness always bears God's image and likeness within themselves, as does every human being. Moreover, they possess the inalienable right to be recognized as images of God and, therefore, to be treated as such."*

As a Catholic priest who has experienced depression, I wholeheartedly agree with this statement. It is worth noting that no one is immune to mental illness; it transcends barriers of culture, religion, race, and nationality. Nevertheless, the harsh reality is that mentally ill individuals are often perceived and treated as lesser humans who have been stripped of their humanity. The stigma associated with mental illness can be more debilitating than the illness itself.

"Did you know that one in five adults suffer from mental illnesses? While this statistic may seem high and alarming, mental illness, like many other disabilities, is often categorized as an "invisible disorder." Many individuals suffer in silence due to the stigma affiliated with mental health diagnoses. Historically, the Catholic Church has not always addressed mental illness. Still, we are called by Jesus to recognize and support those who are suffering among us and accompany them on their journey." (Pastoral statement by the US Catholic Bishops on persons with Disabilities, 1976)

On February 11, 2006, World Day of the Sick, Pope Benedict XVI stated: *"I encourage the efforts of those who strive to ensure that all mentally ill people have access to necessary forms of care and treatment. Unfortunately, in many parts of the world, services for these individuals are lacking, inadequate, or in a state of decay. Their social context does not always accept the mentally ill with their limitations, making it even more challenging to secure the human and financial resources that are needed."*

It could be argued that the most significant barrier to the healing and recovery of individuals with mental illness is the fear rooted in ignorance and the pervasive myths surrounding these conditions, and this factor of fear and ignorance is particularly prevalent in cultures in Nigeria. Many Nigerians are plunged into depression or other mental health challenges as a result of the country's prevailing political and economic instability, exposure to violence, and rising rates of poverty and unemployment.

In my personal journey with depression, I have realized that the onset can be so insidious that you may not even know you are depressed. You begin to drift into a dark pit of self-pity, guilt, feelings of worthlessness, anger, self-resentment, anxiety, withdrawal, loss of interest in social life, and loss of sleep (insomnia). You may even find yourself chronically sad, often without knowing how you arrived at that point.

In Nigeria, discussions and topics about mental health are often stifled by ignorance and stigma, causing many individuals to suffer in silence rather than speak out about the ordeal they are going through. This mismanagement of mental health issues can lead to even greater distress.

One common mistake many in Nigeria make, influenced by cultural or religious points of view, is to 'spiritualize' mentally ill cases. Mental health illness is poorly understood, leading to situations where individuals are chained and confined in unorthodox facilities across the country, including traditional healing and religious centers, rather than receiving appropriate medical care.

As a Church, we are called to break down these barriers of misunderstanding and stigma, to foster a compassionate and supportive environment for those grappling with mental health challenges, and to advocate for the care and treatment that every person deserves.

SPIRITUALIZING MENTAL ILLNESS

Once upon a time, in some areas of Nigeria, the birth of twins was considered taboo and viewed as an evil omen; lacking understanding, communities often abandoned twin infants in the forest. Thankfully, today's narrative has changed significantly. With increased education and awareness, many have come to understand the physiology of having twins and now celebrate their birth as blessings rather than curses.

This transformation highlights a typical human response: fear of the unknown. This fear is especially relevant in the context of mental illnesses, which are often invisible ailments of the mind. Unlike physical conditions that can be diagnosed through tangible symptoms, mental health issues frequently elude recognition and understanding, leading to misconceptions that they are spiritual afflictions.

A prevalent mistake among some religious leaders, including priests, pastors, and Muslim clerics in Nigeria, is the hasty conclusion that people with such illnesses need "spiritual deliverance." This often results in the neglect of proper medical diagnosis and treatment, leaving individuals trapped in their suffering and subjected to endless prayers that fail to address their underlying issues. This cycle of misunderstanding exacerbates the stigma surrounding mental illness, perpetuated by a cloud of ignorance.

As a Catholic Priest of the Roman Rite, I can personally attest to the importance of seeking professional help. During my own experience with clinical depression and anxiety, I was prompted to consult a psychiatrist for a comprehensive assessment. At the end of our first meeting, he confirmed that I was suffering from depression because I exhibited almost all the symptoms (insomnia, self-pity, withdrawal syndrome, loss of appetite, loss of interest in normal daily activities, sense of guilt, self-resentment, suicidal thoughts, feelings of sadness, lack of motivation, poor understanding of hygiene, and anger). My anxiety about my insomnia only intensified the situation; the more I worried, the more elusive sleep became, and no remedy seemed effective.

After diagnosing my depression, the Doctor recommended a series of therapeutic activities and prescribed an antidepressant medication, which I took for a period of time. At the same time, I participated in a psycho-spiritual retreat at the Institute of Consecrated Life in West Africa (InCLA) in Abuja, FCT.

This combination of medical treatment and psycho-spiritual guidance enabled me to reclaim my life. Today, I can confidently say that I am fully recovered, feeling more vibrant and energetic than ever before. I attribute my healing to God, facilitated by the expertise of a qualified doctor and the support of a seasoned psycho-spiritual counselor.

The Catholic Church embodies the principles of FAITH and REASON (*fides et ratio*). Both reason and faith are divine gifts from God that should coexist harmoniously. Now, more than ever, there is a need to understand that science and faith are two sides of the same coin. Just as one would seek medical attention for physical ailments like typhoid fever or malaria, it is equally important to pursue proper medical and spiritual care for mental health issues.

As a priest, I would never suggest that anyone suffering from a physical illness should rely solely on prayer; instead, I would advise and assist the person in seeking medical attention while also providing spiritual support. If this approach is deemed acceptable for physical illnesses, such as typhoid fever and malaria, why should it be any different for mental health conditions? It's time to break the stigma, embrace understanding, and advocate for a holistic approach to health that encompasses both body and mind.

WHAT DOES THE CATHOLIC CHURCH TEACH ABOUT MENTAL HEALTH?

"The Dignity of Every Human Being and the Call to Compassion."

The conviction that every human being, regardless of what ailment they suffer, is created in the image and likeness of God (Genesis 1: 27) serves as a foundational pillar of Christian anthropology. We are called to love one another "as another self" *(Gaudium et Spes, 27).*

Pope Saint John Paul II particularly emphasized that all who suffer from mental illness are equally made in the image and likeness of God and deserving of our love and respect. In addition, they 'always' have the inalienable right not only to be considered as images of God and, therefore, as persons but also to be treated with the dignity that this entails.

Furthermore, we must remember that Christ is present in those who are sick as the gospel of Matthew reminds us, *"I was sick, and you visited me."* (Matthew 25:36). So, as Catholic Christians, we are called to treat all who are ill (whether physically or mentally) as if they were Christ Himself. Pope Saint John Paul II reinforced this notion: *"Well, Christ took all human suffering upon Himself, including mental illness. Yes, even this affliction, which may seem the most absurd and incomprehensible, configures the sick person to Christ and allows them to share in His redeeming passion."*

According to the social teaching of the Catholic Church, access to basic healthcare is not only a fundamental right but also the responsibility of everyone and an essential element of the common good (*Compendium of the Social Doctrine of the Church, 166*).

Pope St. John Paul II urged Christians to engage in compassionate care for our sisters and brothers in need, emphasizing that *"The role of those who care for depressed persons and who do not have a specifically therapeutic task consists above all in helping them to rediscover their self-esteem, confidence in their own abilities, interest in the future, the desire to live. It is therefore important to stretch out a hand to the sick, to make them perceive the tenderness of God, to integrate them into a community of faith and life in which they can feel accepted, understood, supported, and respected in a world in which they can love and be loved."*

Pope Benedict XVI dedicated the 14th World Day of the sick in 2006 to those who have mental illness. In his message for that day, he stated: *"On this occasion, the Church intends to bow down over those who suffer with special concern, calling public attention to the problems connected with mental disturbance that now afflicts one-fifth of humanity and constitutes a real social-health care emergency...."*

He called for a new and better approach to mental health treatment—one that not only provides better medical care but also recognizes the inherent dignity of individuals experiencing mental health challenges. Additionally, he expressed hope that the wider community would be more understanding and show support for people with mental health issues, as well as for those who care for them, many of whom are family members or volunteers who provide care without compensation.

In summary, the call to recognize the dignity of all individuals, especially those facing mental health challenges, is a profound aspect of our Christian faith. It compels us to advocate for better healthcare access and support and embody Christ's love and compassion in our interactions with those who suffer.

THE NEED FOR PSYCHO-SPIRITUAL COUNSELING

My own journey toward healing took a transformative turn when I met Fr. Joel Nkongolo, CMF, a psycho-spiritual counselor at the Institute of Consecrated Life in West Africa (InCLA). At that time, I confided in him about the overwhelming despair that had engulfed me, expressing how I struggled to pray and maintain my faith. I described a profound sense of numbness and emptiness as if the vibrancy of life had drained away from me.

Despite being a Catholic priest for over thirteen years and being well-versed in spiritual teachings, biblical references, and discussions about grace and mercy, I questioned, "What could he possibly say that I haven't heard before?" Yet, when he spoke, he offered a profound insight that resonated with me on a level I had never experienced: "Fr. Andrew, you have experienced the DEATH of your false self; from this point onward, you are about to begin the journey toward your TRUE SELF."

His words struck a deep chord within me, opening my heart to a realization I had never considered. He elaborated that all along, my life had been built upon my EGO-MIND—the false self—rooted in three fundamental areas: (1) affection and esteem, (2) security and survival, and (3) power and control.

Through this psycho-spiritual counseling, Fr Joel guided me on a journey toward the awakening of my true self, often referred to as 'CONSCIOUSNESS.' The true self exists apart from the psychological mind, or what is known as the EGO-MIND, and it is usually the collapse of the EGO-MIND or false self that leads to mental breakdowns. The death of this unconscious false self can give rise to feelings of depression, anxiety, and despair.

This holistic counseling method combines psychological principles with spiritual awareness, offering individuals a framework to explore their mental health and emotional well-being within the context of their cultural and spiritual beliefs. The psychospiritual includes uniting the intellect, soul, and spirit, discovering one's spiritual calling, searching for the meaning of life, or contacting one's true nature.

In Nigeria, it is increasingly recognized as a vital approach to addressing the pervasive issue of burnout, particularly among professionals and caregivers in high-stress environments. In a country where the pressures of daily life, economic challenges, and societal expectations often lead to chronic stress and emotional exhaustion, psychospiritual counseling provides a safe space for individuals to reflect on their experiences, seek meaning, and reconnect with their inner selves.

This approach fosters resilience by integrating traditional healing practices with contemporary psychological techniques. It empowers individuals to navigate the complexities of their lives, ultimately promoting a more balanced and fulfilling existence.

According to Fr George Ehusani - a Catholic Priest working in the Archdiocese of Abuja, Nigeria, and founder of the Psycho-Spiritual Institute (PSI), a Catholic entity that specializes in psycho-trauma healing - he emphasizes the urgent need for psycho-spiritual support in Nigeria owing to the country's political and economic instability that has plunged many into depression and other forms of mental challenges. This offers a path to not only cope with mental health issues but also to rediscover the authentic self, allowing for a deeper connection with God, oneself, and others.

Reflections

1. What lessons have you learned about the importance of advocating for your own health?

2. How can the stigma associated with mental illness be reduced or curbed?

3. Has faith and spirituality ever played a role in your mental health journey?

4. How did it change your perspective on life and your priorities?

6

Chapter Six

THE ROAD TO RECOVERY

"Even the darkest nights will end, and the
Sun will rise again"
- **Victor Hugo.**

I often find myself reflecting on when my journey toward recovery truly began. It is a concept that feels insidious and slippery—much like trying to pinpoint the exact moment my illness took hold of me. One significant turning point came when I realized that, despite being a doctor, I was not the only person in the entire world who felt ill on the inside while appearing perfectly healthy on the outside.

Meeting individuals like Bridget, Dr Abah, and Father Andrew Sule rekindled a flicker of hope within me; sometimes, that is all one needs—hope. Father Andrew Sule spoke about the death of the false self and the journey toward discovering the true self during recovery. Bridget once said to me, "You will not die; however, if you don't seek to get better, you risk living a miserable life." In my experience, I have witnessed countless people who are alive yet not truly living.

The primary reason I am writing this book is to offer hope to anyone going through anxiety, depression, or even suicidal thoughts; there is hope, and though I may sound like a preacher, I speak from a place of understanding.

The road to recovery was anything but easy—I was stuck on medication to sleep and anxiety for over a year, and gradually, I started going out for walks with my wife. At first, even the thought of leaving the house triggered panic attacks, as if everyone could see my suffering. Still, when I go to church, my wife would sit next to me, holding my hand, gently wiping the beads of sweat that formed during my moments of anxiety with a handkerchief.

My body did not respond well to the idea of going outside, preferring to stay indoors, wallowing in self-pity. Yet, with time, I began to rediscover small joys, remember things again, and even sleep for two to three hours a night—what a revelation!

My phone, which had been switched off for so long, was finally turned back on, revealing that calls had ceased; however, my family remained steadfast, reaching out to me occasionally, and they were instrumental in my recovery. I will always be grateful to my dear sister, Mrs. Maureen Ebigbeyi, and my sister-in-law, Mrs. Eunice Ochigbano, who stood by me during those darkest days, feeling our pain deeply.

Despite my reluctance, my unwavering wife, Ehi, took it upon herself to reach out to a few close friends from my past; I'm so thankful she didn't heed my wishes to keep my struggles private.

Odion Omofoman, my best friend from high school and my best man at my wedding in 2008 came to visit. When I confided in him about not sleeping for three months, he remarked, "Your brain must have been fried, man." Another friend, Osagie, was sent by our high school group to check in on me. He was evidently relieved I wasn't "sick" in the conventional sense, yet he still sought to understand what was wrong.

During our extended medical school years lasting 6-8 years due to prolonged labor union strikes by University lecturers—Ogbeide Evbuomwan and I developed a mutual respect for each other. We formed a close friendship, sitting next to each other for nearly every examination because our surnames both started with the letter 'E' and similar adjoining letters. I was honored to be his best man at his wedding, too.

Although he and his family had moved to the UK, he called me every day for two weeks just to talk. Surprisingly, Ogbeide had also suffered minor depression when he moved to the UK, and our conversations became a source of solace for both of us.

As time passed, Ehi began to see glimpses of her old husband returning, with occasional bursts of laughter when I was on the phone. I think she took this as a sign from God and continued to ring up more friends, including my old cycling buddies from the now famous "Abuja ChainGang" cycling club. She even went as far as orchestrating a surprise birthday party with my cycling buddies. This incredible experience brought a smile to my face and sparked laughter within me, creating moments of joy that I had long thought were lost.

People often question whether depression is a genuine experience, and they may wonder how someone can feel such profound unhappiness that they contemplate ending their life. My thoughts might have been similar if I had not walked that path myself. I still remember a friend once saying during a cycling trip, "Depression only happens to weak people." If only he knew the truth behind those words.

In January 2022, Deborah Odoh introduced me to an online course offered by the University of Washington called "Well-Being for Health Professionals." Spanning six weeks, the course provided a fresh perspective on enhancing overall well-being, focusing on three key ingredients: movement (or exercise), breathing (or meditation), and giving back (or charity).

By March 2022, that is thirteen months after I first fell ill, I resumed work in a new position as I understood that I needed help in this role. I also recognized that I needed to approach my job differently, unlike before, as my priorities had experienced a paradigm shift.

My heart rate was almost normal, and I could sleep for about three hours without medication. Though I still had some challenges with memory retention, I was confident it would improve over time, and I anticipated a positive comeback after a few months on the job.

To help with my transition, I enlisted someone to take meeting notes, fearing I might forget important details—but gradually, my memory began to function properly. My outlook on life had fundamentally changed, and as the saying goes, "What does not kill you, makes you stronger." Well, in my case, it felt more like "When one doesn't succeed in extinguishing oneself, one may succeed in reinventing oneself."

I soon realized that many people were going through various phases or degrees of burnout, so I decided to share my experiences with organizations and companies. In October 2022, I co-hosted my first webinar on burnout alongside Bridget for my former organization. What began as a one-hour presentation unexpectedly extended beyond two hours, revealing a significant need for support among individuals grappling with undiagnosed mental health challenges.

Since then, we have delivered this talk at numerous meetings and conferences, both locally and internationally. At every event, at least one person often reaches out afterward to express gratitude or share a personal story, such as, "That's what I think caused my uncle's passing."

During one live webinar, a participant asked, "How do you know this will not reoccur again? How can you stop this from reoccurring? I usually smile at such questions, appreciating their depths. Now, I take deliberate and strategic steps to protect my mental health by delegating work and maintaining a clear distinction between work and personal time. I have learned the importance of not bringing work home every night and weekend—after all, the world won't collapse if I don't.

My first step was ensuring my entire team respected boundaries between work and personal life, including email etiquette. However, one challenge to this approach is that toxic work culture has become institutionalized in most work environments, fueled by a "do or die" mentality. I strive to foster a healthier work environment, but it requires consistent effort and collective commitment; in addition, I have come to truly appreciate the importance of finding time for rest.

Dr Saundra Dalton-Smith identifies seven types of rest that I strive to incorporate into my lifestyle:

1. **Physical Rest:** The first type of rest we need is physical rest, which can be either passive or active. The "passive physical rest" includes sleeping and napping, while "active physical rest" involves restorative activities such as yoga, stretching, and massage therapy that improve the body's circulation and flexibility. We should ensure restful sleep—aiming for at least seven hours. In contrast, during my burnout experience, I struggled to achieve this for three months.

2. **Mental Rest:** Do you start your workday with a large cup of coffee? Are you often irritable, forgetful, and have difficulty concentrating? Do racing thoughts from the day keep you awake when you lie down to sleep at night? Even after sleeping seven to eight hours, do you wake up feeling unrested? If so, you may be experiencing a mental rest deficit, and it's crucial to take time to clear your mind.

I enjoy listening to all genres of music, including *Burna Boy's* "*Dangote,*" while driving to the office, and I also love catching up with the latest Netflix top 10 movies. Scheduling short breaks every two hours during your workday can help you slow down; additionally, keeping a notepad by your bed to jot down nagging thoughts can be beneficial.

3. **Sensory Rest:** Finding sensory rest can be challenging in our age of information overload from our digital devices. Bright lights, computer screens, background noise, and multiple

conversations, whether in an office or on Zoom calls, can cause our senses to feel overwhelmed.

Nonetheless, we must remember that there was a time when we had healthy lives before these "smart" devices came into existence. Now, I make it a point of duty to leave my work laptop at the office when going home and only address emergency work-related calls on weekends

4. **Social Rest**: Nurturing positive relationships is vital for recharging our social batteries. This implies that it is essential to differentiate between relationships that revive us and those that drain our energy. My experiences have taught me the importance of prioritizing family, which should always come first.

5. **Emotional Rest**: Let's talk about someone we all know—the friend who everyone believes is the nicest person ever. This is the person everyone turns to for help, the one you would call when you need a favor; even if they are not eager to help, you know they will give you a reluctant "Yes" instead of a straightforward "No." However, when this friend is left alone, they often feel unappreciated and taken advantage of. They need emotional rest, which means having the time and space to express their feelings honestly and to stop constantly trying to please others.

Emotional rest also requires the courage to be genuine; a person who has had this rest can answer the question "How are you today?" with a sincere "I'm not okay," and feel comfortable sharing things that usually remain unspoken.

It is crucial to be genuine when expressing our emotions and avoid bottling things up because, as for me, I don't whitewash situations, and I utilize emotional intelligence skills to help manage my team.

6. **Spiritual Rest**: The final type of rest allows us to connect beyond the physical and mental realms, fostering a deep sense of belonging, love, acceptance, and purpose. Father Sule discusses this concept extensively in his book. We all need to find our true purpose and sense of belonging in life—Personally, I find philanthropic activities to be spiritually fulfilling.

7. **Creative Rest**: This type of rest is vital for anyone who must solve problems or brainstorm new ideas. Some people like my former self would travel on vacations and spend the entire time glued to their laptops searching for deals on some high street instead of relaxing.

I have learned the importance of getting creative rest to rejuvenate and reboot our system. This does not have to be on an exotic Island or Kenyan resort; sometimes, a simple getaway can suffice. My first true restful vacation after over 46 years of my life was a four-day holiday at a Beach Island in Lagos, and since then, I have made sure to plan at least one every year.

Dr Saundra's belief is that restoring balance in all these areas is essential to curing your "rest deficit" and attaining better mental health. Through this journey, I learned that recovery is not just about overcoming illness; it's also about rediscovering the connections and joys in life that make it meaningful. While the path may be fraught with challenges, it is also illuminated by the support of loved ones and the hope that fuels our healing.

I acknowledge that I am still a work in progress and grateful for every day, as it remains a gift. It would be impossible to recount my recovery journey without recognizing the unwavering support of my lovely wife, Ehigocho, and my son, Oritseweyinmi. They witnessed the turmoil unfold, with their lives torn apart before their very eyes, and stood by me through it all—they are the true heroes of my story. You both are simply the best!!

Reflections

1. What boundaries do you currently have between your work and personal life?

2. Are there areas where you could improve?

3. In what ways can you contribute to creating a healthier work environment for yourself and your colleagues?

4. What have you learned about the importance of self-care and stress management?

5. What specific actions will you commit to prioritize your mental well-being in the coming weeks or months?

Conclusion

This book has illuminated the complex landscape of burnout, examining its symptoms—such as chronic fatigue, emotional detachment, and a pervasive sense of inadequacy—that can leave individuals feeling drained and isolated.

We explored the various causes of burnout, from overwhelming workloads and lack of support to societal pressures that demand perfection and relentless productivity. These factors contribute not only to personal suffering but also to a culture of stigmatization that discourages open discussions about mental health.

Recognizing and addressing these symptoms and causes is essential for healing, and we have discussed various actionable solutions. Implementing self-care practices like mindfulness and exercise, seeking professional help, and advocating for systemic changes in our workplaces can significantly alleviate the burden of burnout.

It's crucial to foster environments where dialogue about mental health is encouraged, allowing individuals to share their experiences without fear of judgment.

As you close this book, I encourage you to reflect on your own experiences and consider the steps you can take—both individually and collectively—to address burnout. Remember, acknowledging burnout is not a sign of weakness but a courageous act of self-awareness.

Together, we can break the silence, challenge the stigma, and pave the way for a healthier, more compassionate approach to well-being. Let this be the beginning of a journey toward resilience, connection, and a renewed sense of purpose.

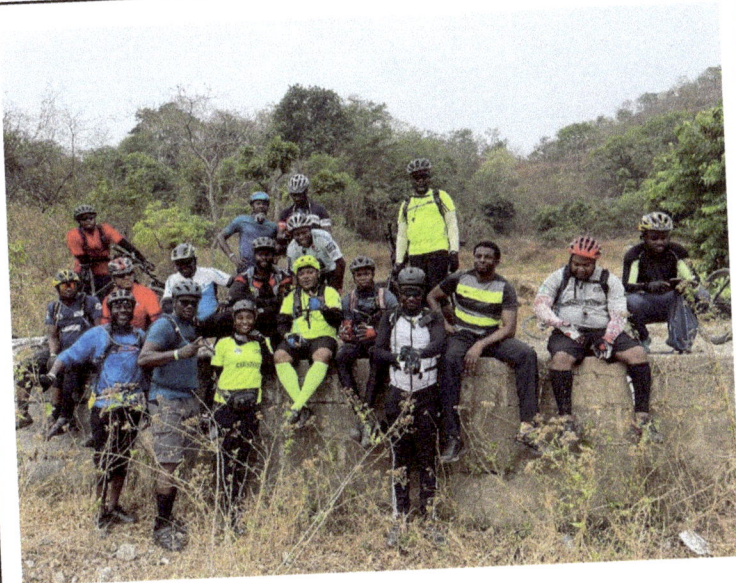

picture represents my first bicycle ride after my recovery from burnout